Chocolate

Treat Yourself to a Healthy Heart

Barbara Wexler, MPH

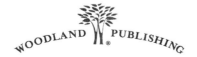

Copyright © 2008 by Barbara Wexler

All rights reserved. No part of this publication may be reproduced, stored in retrieval system, or transmitted in any form without the prior written permission of the copyright owner.

For permissions, ordering information, or bulk quantity discounts, contact: Woodland Publishing, 448 East 800 North, Orem, Utah 84097

Visit our Web site: www.woodlandpublishing.com
Toll-free number: (800) 777-BOOK (2665)

The information in this book is for educational purposes only and is not recommended as a means of diagnosing or treating an illness. All matters concerning physical and mental health should be supervised by a health practitioner knowledgeable in treating that particular condition. Neither the publisher nor the author directly or indirectly dispenses medical advice, nor do they prescribe any remedies or assume any responsibility for those who choose to treat themselves.

Cataloging-in-Publication data is available from the Library of Congress.

ISBN: 978-1-58054-112-1

Printed in the United States of America

Contents

Bittersweet Bliss   5
A Rich History   5
Craving Chocolate?   6
Sidebar: Is Chocolate Better Than Sex?   9
Chocolate Promotes a Positive Outlook   10
And Packs a Nutritional Punch   11
But Is It a Health Food?   12
Chocolate Lowers Blood Pressure   13
And Reduces the Risk of Heart Disease   14
All About Antioxidants   15
Sidebar: A Delicious Concept   17
Hearts and Sales Soar   17
Bittersweet, Dark or Milk?   18
Myths About Chocolate Dispelled   20
Sidebar: How to Make Chocolate
   in 16 Not-So-Easy Steps   21
References   29

Bittersweet Bliss

I love you more than chocolate itself.
—Sandra Boynton

When Joseph Campbell, the renowned American professor of mythology and comparative religion, proclaimed that the secret of life was to follow your bliss, chocolate lovers around the world smiled knowingly—they were already way ahead of the curve. Recent scientific research has shown that, in addition to other mood- and health-enhancing compounds, chocolate contains a class of psychoactive chemicals called anandamides, or "bliss compounds" (the term has its roots in the ancient Sanskrit word *ananda,* meaning "bliss"—a state of spiritual perfection that transcends the ordinary limitations of mind and body).

Before you dismiss that description as being a little extreme for chocolate, you may want to consider the early history of chocolate, and the fact that it was at times reserved exclusively for emperors, priests and warriors.

A Rich History

The cacao tree, from which chocolate is derived, is native to Central and South America. Scholars believe that the first cacao plants probably appeared about 15,000 years ago in the area around modern Venezuela. Today, cacao is cultivated in the Caribbean, Africa, Southeast Asia and the South Pacific Islands of Samoa and New Guinea.

Archaeologists have recently discovered traces of chocolate in ceramic pots at least 2,600 years old—artifacts of the mysterious Olmec culture of southern Mexico and Central America. The later Mayan and Aztec cultures used chocolate extensively, although ancient chocolate was a far cry from today's sweet foil-wrapped bars and cream-filled truffles. Traditionally, chocolate was consumed as a fermented beverage called *xocolatl*—a heady brew made of cacao beans, hot chili and corn.

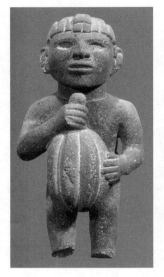

The Aztecs prized chocolate so highly that they used cacao beans—the seed from which all chocolate is made—as currency. A dozen beans were good for an unforgettable night with a courtesan and 100 beans could purchase a household slave for life. When the Spanish conquistador Hernán Cortés defeated the emperor Moctezuma in 1519, instead of a palace filled with gold and jewels he found storehouses filled with chocolate. It is estimated that the upkeep of Moctezuma's royal household cost as much as of 12 *million* cacao beans every year!

The ancient Mesoamericans weren't the only people to appreciate chocolate's blissful nature. The eighteenth-century Swedish botanist and physician Carolus Linnaeus, father of modern scientific nomenclature, dubbed the cacao plant *Theobroma cacao*—literally, "food of the gods." Linnaeus and his contemporaries enthusiastically integrated chocolate into their medical practices; in 1792 the physician Alexander Peter Buchan recommended that women in labor be given chocolate to prevent fainting brought on by blood loss.

Craving Chocolate?

Strength is the capacity to break a chocolate bar into four pieces with your bare hands—and then eat just one of the pieces.

—Judith Viorst

Nearly everyone loves chocolate; on average, the Swiss consume more than 21 pounds of chocolate per person per year, while the Belgians and the British eat about 16 pounds annually. In the United States, the average adult consumes nearly 12 pounds of chocolate per year—about one pound per month, or a chocolate bar every other day.

For many people, nothing satisfies a sweet tooth as well as chocolate. Its rich, intense flavor and creamy texture make chocolate irresistibly deli ous—about 15 percent of men and more than 40 percent of women report chocolate cravings. But the addictive quality of chocolate—the reason it evokes such powerful cravings—may rest in chocolate's ability to stimulate psychoactive chemicals in the brain.

Chocolate contains tryptophan, a chemical the brain uses to make serotonin (which acts as an antidepressant); phenylethylamine, which promotes feelings of giddiness, excitement and attraction; and anandamide, which binds to the cannabinoid receptor (the same receptor that binds delta-9-tetrahydrocannabinol [THC], the active ingredient in marijuana). Chocolate also contains and stimulates the secretion of many other neurochemicals, including endorphins—the pleasure-producing feel-good chemicals in the brain. Let's consider how the actions of some of these chemicals help improve mood and provide an overall sense of well-being.

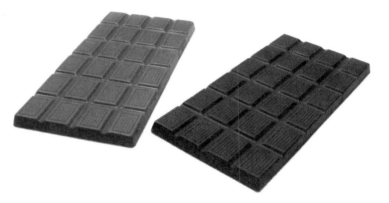

The Serenity of Serotonin

Nerve cells talk to one another through electrical impulses, and neurotransmitters shape and direct their communication by amplifying, relaying, blocking and modulating nervous system messages. Serotonin is one of the most important neurotransmitters and has been identified as a key regulator of mood, sleep, sexuality and appetite. Many antidepressant drugs—selective serotonin reuptake inhibitors (SSRIs) like Prozac, Zoloft and Paxil—work by blocking the body's resorption of serotonin, effectively keeping each molecule in play for a longer period of time.

It's tempting to think that we can relieve our stress, anxiety or depression by taking extra serotonin in the form of a pill. And it may be even more tempting to think that we can substitute a chocolate truffle for daily dose of antidepressant! Unfortunately, the serotonin molecu doesn't pass through the protective barrier between the bloodstream a the brain. Any serotonin we consume directly will simply be broken dow without doing us any good.

However, consuming the nutritional precursors of serotonin ca influence the body's level of serotonin. Serotonin is synthesized from tl amino acid L-tryptophan, and many people report that taking L-trypte phan brightens their mood, improves their quality of sleep, helps the to resist depression and anxiety and relieves many symptoms of stres Since chocolate contains tryptophan, it can boost serotonin productio which can in turn generate feelings of satisfaction, contentment ar even elation.

Interestingly, the chocolate cravings some women experience in tl days preceding menstruation may be explained by fluctuations in sere tonin. Ecco Bella, a retailer of designer chocolates, has capitalized on th potential link between PMS and chocolate cravings; the label of tl Women's Wonder Bar encourages women to "take sweet revenge c PMS!"

The Excitement of Phenylethylamine

Phenylethylamine is a neurotransmitter that occurs naturally in choce late and the oil derived from bitter almonds. Its structure and pharmace logical properties are similar to those of amphetamine—phenylethy amine stimulates a rush of pleasurable feelings such as giddy joy, excite ment and euphoria. It has been said that phenylethylamine is to passio what endorphins are to love because phenylethylamine stimulates tl brain's pleasure centers and levels of the neurotransmitter rise durir sexual activity and peak at orgasm.

Naturally, this raises the question of the connection between chocola and sex. Some women have compared the experience of eating chocola to sexual passion. Fewer men than women describe chocolate this way– but that wasn't always the case. Chocolate has a long history as a repute aphrodisiac; purportedly, the Aztec emperor Moctezuma drank 50 gol lets of chocolate a day to enhance his sexual prowess, and the legendar lover Giacomo Casanova ate chocolate before pursuing his conquests.

Researchers in the Netherlands may have uncovered the explanatio for the gender difference in chocolate cravings. They performed a study i which subjects fasted overnight and were then scanned using functional magnetic resonance imaging while tasting chocolate milk—before and after eating chocolate—until they were completely satiated. The researchers discovered that the taste of chocolate activated different parts of the brain in men and women. Interestingly, the circuits in the brain that respond to sex and music also respond to chocolate.

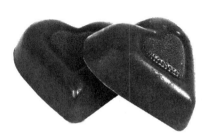

Is Chocolate Better than Sex?

There is no question that chocolate is one of the world's most delicious and desirable foods, but is it better than sex? In a recent survey, more than half of the women interviewed said that they would generally choose chocolate over sex. (Of course, that's a tad ironic, since a recent study in Italy found that women who regularly consumed chocolate reported having more satisfying sex lives than their chocolate-deprived counterparts.) Whatever your thoughts on the subject, it's clear that chocolate is very much an object of desire in and of itself. As we've observed, chocolate can generate intense cravings comparable to the effects of narcotics and mind-altering drugs.

The Natural High of Anandamide

Anandamide is among the most psychoactive substances in chocolate. Chocolate also contains two chemicals known to slow the breakdown of anandamide, prolonging its action in the brain. Since anandamide targets the same brain structures as THC (the active ingredient in marijuana), some people believe it contributes to the "high" many people report after eating chocolate.

But many researchers question whether the amount of anandamide in chocolate is sufficient to produce any effect at all. These researchers assert that it would require consumption of huge amounts of chocolate—pounds at a time—to generate any perceptible difference in mood.

Endorphins to Relieve Pain and Elevate Mood

Eating chocolate triggers the release of endorphins, the body's endogenous (self-produced) opiates. Endorphins are chemically comparable to morphine, a substance derived from opium that elevates mood and reduces pain (the term *endorphin* means "endogenous morphine"). Endorphins are amino acid residues that occur naturally in the brain; they work by binding to opiate receptors and have potent pain-relieving properties. The endorphins released in response to tasting chocolate probably contribute to the warm inner glow and deep satisfaction reported by chocolate lovers.

Chocolate Promotes a Positive Outlook

In one German study, researchers fed 37 healthy women a chocolate bar, an apple or nothing at all. The researchers then assessed the women's emotional states 15, 30, 60 and 90 minutes after eating. The results showed that while both chocolate and apples reduced hunger and elevated mood, the effects of the chocolate were stronger. Eating chocolate was also followed by joy (and, in some women, by guilt).

Some of the same researchers then tested two hypotheses about the effects of chocolate on mood: first, that eating a piece of chocolate immediately improves negative, but not positive or neutral, mood; and second, that this effect is largely due to chocolate's taste. They found that eating chocolate improved negative mood while having only marginal effects—if any at all—on neutral and positive mood. Negative mood was improved only after eating tasty—as opposed to tasteless—chocolate.

But the study noted that the mood improvement was short-lived, lasting only about three minutes. (The impulse to scarf down a chocolate bar when you're feeling blue may be a good one—as long as you don't expect more than a few minutes' reprieve from the blues!) The researchers concluded that eating a small amount of sweet food improves a negative mood state immediately and selectively, and that this effect of chocolate is largely due to the chocolate's taste.

And Packs a Nutritional Punch

Chocolate is certainly not junk food—it contains a number of important nutrients. One ounce (28.35 grams) of dark chocolate contains 136 calories 1.19 grams of protein, 8.51 grams of fat, 9 mg of calcium, 33 mg of magnesium, 37 mg of phosphorus, 103 mg of potassium and 18 mg of caffeine. Chocolate also delivers vitamins B1, B2, D and E.

Although chocolate does contain fat (some of it saturated), dark chocolate has been shown to exert a beneficial effect on blood cholesterol. The fat in dark chocolate is largely stearic acid and oleic acid. Stearic acid is a saturated fat, but unlike most saturated fats it does not raise blood cholesterol levels. Oleic acid, a monounsaturated fat, does not raise cholesterol and may even reduce it. And chocolate is made without using hydrogenated or partially hydrogenated oils, which are known to increase cholesterol levels. But be careful to avoid chocolate candies such as bonbons and candy bars that contain ingredients other than chocolate, some of which may include hydrogenated and partially hydrogenated oils.

Dark chocolate is a potent source of two bioflavonoids—procyanidins and epicatechins. Bioflavonoids have been termed natural biological response modifiers because of their ability to adapt and moderate the body's reaction to microbes—allergens, viruses and carcinogens (cancer-causing agents). Bioflavonoids have demonstrated many health benefits, including anti-allergic, anti-inflammatory, antimicrobial and anticancer activity. Bioflavonoids serve as powerful antioxidants, protecting cells against oxidative stress and free-radical damage. Laboratory research has even demonstrated that some bioflavonoids suppress tumor growth.

But Is It a Health Food?

The superiority of chocolate, both for health and nourishment, will soon give it the same preference over tea and coffee in America which it has in Spain.
—THOMAS JEFFERSON

Because of chocolate's calorie content, it's difficult to support the claim that chocolate is the ultimate diet food. But chocolate definitely isn't junk food and its calories certainly aren't empty. Although the average chocolate bar contains about 250 calories, even calorie counters can enjoy a small amount of chocolate as an occasional treat. Some dieters assert that high-quality dark chocolate (70 percent cocoa or more) is so rich and delicious that just a small portion satisfies them and quells the urge to overindulge in other sweets.

Believe it or not, a dark chocolate bar actually packs a greater antioxidant punch than a bowl of blueberries or a cup of tea. (Per capita, chocolate is the third highest daily source of dietary antioxidants in the United States.) Not surprisingly, research has linked antioxidant-rich dark chocolate to many health benefits.

In one animal study of heart disease, researchers found that daily cocoa powder (at a dose equivalent in humans to two bars of dark chocolate) significantly inhibited atherosclerosis; lowered cholesterol, low-density lipoprotein and triglycerides; raised high-density lipoprotein and protected lower-density lipoproteins from oxidation.

One study found that eating 3.5 ounces of dark chocolate raised the levels of polyphenols (health-promoting phytochemicals) in the blood by nearly 20 percent. Another reported that eating the same amount of dark chocolate every day for two weeks reduced blood pressure in persons with high blood pressure.

In another study, researchers fed different types of chocolate to healthy men and women aged 25 to 35. Each day, the subjects ate either 100 grams of dark chocolate by itself, 100 grams of dark chocolate with a small glass of whole milk, or 200 grams of milk chocolate. One hour after eating the chocolate, the subjects who ate dark chocolate alone had the most antioxidants in their blood and the highest levels of epicatechins. The milk chocolate eaters had the lowest levels of epicatechins.

Despite these health benefits, most nutritionists don't recommend getting all—or even many—of your daily antioxidants from dark chocolate; if you do, you'll also get a hefty serving of sugar, saturated fat and calories, which could lead to weight gain. And if you gain weight, you'll offset many of the health benefits you gain by consuming antioxidants.

For your health, it's probably best to make chocolate an occasional indulgence. To satisfy your cravings and reap the most benefits, choose dark chocolate over milk chocolate. Dark chocolate contains a higher concentration of cocoa (and antioxidants) than milk chocolate and helps to increase levels of HDL ("good") cholesterol.

Chocolate Lowers Blood Pressure

Recently the media have given considerable attention to the health benefits of tea; but when it comes to reducing blood pressure, chocolate trumps tea, according to research conducted at the University of Cologne Hospital in Germany.

The researchers reviewed the relevant medical literature to compare the blood pressure–lowering effects of cocoa and tea. They found that the reduction in blood pressure among subjects who consumed cocoa products for at least two weeks was in the same range as that of an individual who took prescription drugs commonly prescribed to control high blood pressure. This decrease in blood pressure could reduce the risk of stroke and heart attack by as much as 10 to 20 percent.

The researchers concluded that consumption of foods rich in cocoa may reduce blood pressure, while tea intake appears to have no effect. They speculated that the polyphenols in cocoa may be more bioavailable than those in tea. Both tea and chocolate contain comparable amounts of polyphenols, but the components of those polyphenols differ—cocoa is rich in procyanidins, whereas tea is rich in flavan-3-ols and gallic acid.

The same researchers conducted another study and found that it takes just a small amount of chocolate—less than the amount in two Hershey's

Kisses per day—to lower blood pressure. For 18 weeks the researchers followed 44 otherwise healthy adults, ages 56 to 73, with mild high blood pressure or prehypertension. During this time the subjects were randomly assigned to receive a daily dose of either 6.3 grams of dark chocolate (containing 30 mg of polyphenols) or the same amount of white chocolate (which isn't really chocolate and contains no polyphenols) in addition to their normal diets.

In the dark chocolate group, systolic blood pressure dropped an average of nearly three points, and diastolic blood pressure dropped almost two points. (Population studies estimate that a three-point reduction in systolic blood pressure reduces the risk for stroke, cardiovascular disease and death from all causes by 8 percent, 5 percent and 4 percent, respectively.) In contrast, blood pressure remained unchanged in the white chocolate group. Body weight remained constant in both groups. Although the study was small and must be confirmed by further research, its findings support previous conclusions that ongoing dark chocolate consumption induces chemical changes that help dilate blood vessels and regulate blood pressure. The finding that even small amounts of chocolate can exert powerful health benefits is good news for those who worry about adding too many calories to their diets.

The blood-pressure improvements associated with daily chocolate consumption were similar to those observed among people who adhere to the Dietary Approaches to Stop Hypertension (DASH) diet. And while the DASH diet—which is low in saturated and total fat and rich in fruits, vegetables and low-fat dairy foods—is effective, it is also complicated. It's much easier—and more pleasant—to simply eat a piece of dark chocolate every day!

And Reduces the Risk of Heart Disease

As previously mentioned, chocolate contains bioflavonoids, which are thought to reduce the risk of heart disease at least in part by reducing LDL ("bad") cholesterol and inflammation. Although studies on the relationship between bioflavonoids and heart health have produced mixed results—some show a modest benefit, others report no significant benefit—new research continues to support the heart-health benefits of bioflavonoids.

Recently, researchers scrutinized the diets of 34,489 postmenopausal women who did not have cardiovascular disease to see if bioflavonoid consumption was related to cardiovascular disease risk and mortality. They examined bioflavonoid intake and rates of heart disease over a 16-year period and found that three—anthocyanidins, flavanones, and flavones—were associated with a significantly reduced risk of cardiovascular disease mortality. The researchers also identified dark chocolate, along with apples, pears and red wine, as a specific food linked to reductions in cardiovascular disease.

All About Antioxidants

When certain atoms within the body lose an electron, they become unstable. These unstable atoms—free radicals—are responsible for oxidative stress—the equivalent of rusting in the body. Combating oxidative stress is a nonstop biological process that is vital to our health. While our bodies naturally contain a number of systems that control the ravages of oxidizing radicals, we also receive help from antioxidants (sometimes called free-radical scavengers) that we obtain from our foods. Antioxidants provide the following benefits:

- Enhanced intercellular communication and coordination
- Correction of errors introduced into DNA by toxins
- Enhanced responsiveness of the immune system
- Improved cellular response to essential hormonal signals
- Increased detoxification of potentially cancer-causing substances
- Improved apoptosis (the natural process by which the body rids itself of cancerous and infected cells)
- Better resistance to cardiovascular disease
- Improved bone health and resistance to osteoporosis
- Enhanced eye health (including prevention of macular degeneration and cataracts)

Fresh fruits and vegetables are typically the best source of naturally occurring antioxidants. The strong colors of these living foods actually come from phytonutrient pigments that act as powerful antioxidants. For this reason, nutritionists recommend that we eat a variety of fruits and vegetables of all colors. As we increase our consumption of processed foods and decrease our consumption of fresh fruits and vegetables, we have a greater need to obtain antioxidants from other sources, including other types of foods and nutritional supplements.

Attack of the Killer ORACs

While ORAC might sound like a ravenous beast from *The Lord of the Rings*, it is actually the name of a laboratory procedure that tests a substance's ability to combat the oxidation that takes place inside the body. The ORAC (Oxygen Radical Absorbance Capacity) procedure measures the ability of a substance to neutralize the most common source of oxidative stress in the body, a chemical unit called the peroxyl radical. ORAC testing helps us determine which foods and supplements do the best job of neutralizing potentially harmful free radicals and resisting oxidative stress.

The ORAC test is a wonderful tool; however, consumers should know that ORAC values can be easily manipulated to make products look more appealing and healthful than they really are. A new marketing trend involves skewing ORAC values (for example, by quoting the ORAC value for a whole package of a food product rather than for a reasonable single serving). As the "ORAC wars" heat up in health food marketing, watchdog groups are trying to create guidelines for the ethical and informative use of ORAC data.

Chocolate-Coated Antioxidants

It's been known for some time that chocolate products, especially those made with high levels of cacao, contain an excellent array of natural antioxidants. Consequently, their ORAC values can be quite high. But does a high ORAC value really mean that chocolate is good for you?

One recent study, supported by the American Heart Association and the National Center for Complementary and Alternative Medicine and conducted by the Linus Pauling Institute (at Oregon State University), provided new insight into what chocolate does for us. The researchers' findings read like a good-news/bad-news joke:

Good news: The ORAC values of some of the natural compounds in chocolate, particularly proanthocyanidin, are impressively high.

Bad news: These compounds are not very bioavailable—only a small percentage is actually absorbed into the body.

Good news: A very small amount of proanthocyanidin has a very big beneficial effect. That's because rather than acting like an antioxidant, mopping up damaging free radicals, proanthocyanidin acts like a trigger, switching on natural cellular processes that increase the body's capacity for free-radical cleanup.

Bad news: We don't have an excuse to eat a lot of chocolate for its health benefits—even a small amount will provide enough proanthocyanidin to do the trick!

A Delicious Concept

In 2005, Memorial Hospital in South Bend, Indiana, partnered with the South Bend Chocolate Company to open a chocolate café on the hospital campus. Along with fine chocolates, the Chocolate Café at Memorial serves a range of healthy fare including soups and salads. Supporters observe that, in addition to the acknowledged health benefits of chocolate, the café provides a playful and indulgent environment that acts as a stress reliever for anxious patients, families and hospital personnel (café staff members wear shirts emblazoned with "chocolate therapist" and hats advising that they "will work for chocolate").

By 2007 the café was so successful that Memorial Hospital and the South Bend Chocolate Factory launched a third company, Chocolate Café Medical Ventures Group, to expand the concept across the country. In the future, chocolate cafés may be as common in hospitals as operating rooms!

Hearts (and Sales) Soar

Industry analysts assert that new research characterizing chocolate as a heart-healthy indulgence has led to healthy increases in dark chocolate sales; one study reported an increase of nearly 50 percent from 2003 to

2006. In March 2007, cocoa futures reached a four-year high when dark chocolate sales topped $1.88 billion in the United States.

Chocolate makers have been quick to respond to the demand for healthy chocolate. In 2003, a German confectioner promoted an "anti-aging" chocolate made with dark chocolate, mango and soymilk. In 2006, Mars, Inc., introduced CocoaVia, a line of premium chocolate products marketed as heart-healthy choices. In the same year, the Hershey Company complemented its premium Extra Dark and Cacao Reserve dark chocolate lines by acquiring Dagoba, an organic chocolate brand that not only promotes economic and environmental sustainability but also uses herbs and other natural ingredients to boost the health benefits of its already antioxidant-rich chocolate.

Still, some experts caution against marketing chocolate solely as a health food. Industry analysts warn that this approach could backfire with consumers who prefer to view chocolate as an indulgence rather than as a health food. And nutritionists, many of whom are skeptical of marketing claims that overemphasize chocolate's health benefits, contend that in terms of health, a little chocolate goes a long way. Of course, nutrition alone is not responsible for the chocolate boom—skyrocketing sales can also be attributed to the increasing availability of designer and artisan chocolates with innovative—even exotic—flavor combinations.

Bittersweet, Dark or Milk?

All of the evil that people have thrust upon chocolate is really more deserved by milk chocolate, which is essentially contaminated. The closer you get to a pure chocolate liquor (the chocolate essence ground from roasted cacao beans) the purer it is, the more satisfying it is, the safer it is, and the healthier it is.

—Arnold Ismach
The Darker Side of Chocolate

Milk chocolate, dark chocolate, bittersweet chocolate, chocolate with almonds, chocolate-covered fruit—there are so many delicious choices. In terms of pure pleasure, let your palate be your guide. In terms of nutrition, however, not all chocolate is created equal.

Unsweetened chocolate has 100 percent cacao content and is too bitter to be eaten plain. It is made from ground cocoa nibs and may be natural or Dutch. Dutch cocoa, which is treated with an alkalizing agent to cut its acidity, has a deeper color and a milder flavor than natural, unprocessed cocoa. Dutch cocoa is frequently used for chocolate drinks (such as hot chocolate) because it blends easily with liquids. It is also a common ingredient in chocolate candy, ice cream and baked goods. Although Dutch chocolate is easier to incorporate into food products and beverages, Dutch processing destroys most of the bioflavonoids in cocoa.

Sweet chocolate, commonly called dark chocolate, contains at least 15 percent unsweetened chocolate and less than 12 percent milk solids. Although it has lower cacao content than unsweetened chocolate, dark chocolate may contain as much as 99 percent cacao. Eating dark chocolate with a high concentration of cocoa solids—70 percent or higher—is far and away the best way to satisfy a chocolate craving without consuming too much sugar and saturated fat.

Milk chocolate generally contains at least 10 percent unsweetened chocolate, 12 percent milk solids and about 3 percent milk fat. Its cacao content is relatively low—usually from 30 to 49 percent. White chocolate (which contains no cacao and is really not chocolate at all) is made from cocoa butter—which lends it a subtle, often barely detectable, chocolate flavor—blended with milk solids, lecithin, vanilla and sugar.

Bitter Is Better

Before the addition of sweeteners, emulsifiers and other ingredients, cacao is bitter and grainy. In fact, historically chocolate was used as a savory ingredient rather than a sweet, often seasoned with chili peppers or other strong flavors. It wasn't until modern times that chocolate was transformed into the sweet and creamy confection we know today—and therein lies the rub. Because while chocolate itself contains an incredible wealth of healthful substances, the sugar, fats, milk products and other added ingredients in most chocolate products may eclipse any health benefits. So the next time you feel the need to indulge in a chocolate treat, look for chocolate in its purest, most unprocessed state. Your heart—and your taste buds—will thank you!

Myths About Chocolate Dispelled

Chocolate causes cavities.
Fermentable carbohydrates—which provide food for acid-forming bacteria in the mouth—cause cavities. And while there are fermentable carbohydrates in chocolate, there is also cocoa butter, which coats the teeth and protects them against decay. And unlike other sugary treats, chocolate melts quickly in the mouth, leaving decay-promoting bacteria very little time to adhere to the teeth.

Researchers at Japan's Osaka University have found that the husks of cocoa beans contain an antibacterial agent that fights plaque; however, they concluded that the cavity-fighting action of cocoa bean husks is not sufficient to offset the potential for decay caused by chocolate's high sugar content.

According to researchers at Tulane University, an extract of cocoa powder might be an effective natural alternative to fluoride in toothpaste. It's even possible that cocoa extract will prove more effective than fluoride in preventing cavities. The extract, a white crystalline powder that is chemically comparable to caffeine, helps harden tooth enamel, making teeth more resilient and less susceptible to decay.

While it seems unlikely that chocolate will replace toothpaste in the foreseeable future, it's potential benefits to dental health mean that chocolate probably shouldn't bear too much of the blame for tooth decay.

Chocolate is high in caffeine.
One ounce of milk chocolate contains 6 mg of caffeine—just a little bit more than the amount found in a cup of decaffeinated coffee. One ounce of dark chocolate contains 18 mg of caffeine, or about as much as in a half cup of green tea.

Chocolate causes acne.
The milk solids in many chocolate products may exacerbate acne, but acne isn't caused by chocolate. In fact, the antioxidants in chocolate can actually help to improve the skin's health and appearance.

Chocolate is a common cause of allergic reactions.
True chocolate allergies—allergic reactions to cocoa itself—are actually quite rare. More often people are intolerant of an ingredient in chocolate

or an additive used to prepare it. Potential problem ingredients include soy lecithin, milk, corn syrup, gluten, nuts, flavorings and food coloring.

While chocolate allergies are uncommon, some people are sensitive to naturally occurring chemicals in chocolate like caffeine, theobromine and phenylethylamine. These chemicals may prompt headaches or mood swings in sensitive people, but such reactions are not considered allergies.

How to Make Chocolate in 16 Not-So-Easy Steps

Because chocolate is everywhere in our culture—from supermarket checkout lanes to the kitchens of five-star restaurants—it's pretty easy to take it for granted. And because chocolate can be so inexpensive, it can be a real eye-opener to learn how incredibly complex, difficult and labor-intensive chocolate production is.

Modern chocolate making is a major industry complete with intricate computer-controlled machinery and complex, interdependent processes. But it might surprise you to learn that, as advanced and automated as the technology of chocolate production has become, 90 percent of all the cacao trees from which chocolate is made are still grown on small family farms—usually 12 acres or less—and that the delicate cacao pods are individually harvested and processed by hand.

Why, in the fast-paced twenty-first century, does the cultivation of cacao remain a painstakingly manual process? The answer lies in the economic value and delicacy of the cacao tree itself.

It takes about six years for a new tree to mature and start producing usable seedpods. When fully productive, that tree will only produce enough rich, flavorful seeds to make about two pounds of bittersweet chocolate per year. Cacao growers, even if they could afford modern harvesting machinery, would not be willing to risk the health of their valuable trees, especially since, unlike seasonal crops, cacao trees produce pods continuously. So to protect the trees—and their valuable investment—cacao growers harvest the pods one-by-one in the time-honored fashion.

But the careful hand cultivation of cacao is just the beginning. What follows is a very brief description of the 16 not-so-easy steps required to make chocolate.

Step 1: Picking the pods
The ripe pods of the cacao tree (sometimes called *cabosses*) are gently cut from the tree by hand, usually with a large machete. Each pod contains upwards of 40 cacao beans. A mature tree produces about 30 pods per year, providing about 1,000 usable beans—enough to make approximately two pounds of chocolate.

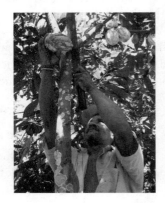

Step 2: Opening the pods
The cacao pods are opened by hand with a machete or a large knife and the beans are removed. In their natural state, cacao beans are surrounded by a sticky white pulp with a strange taste that is both bitter and sweet at the same time. While this pulp does not become part of the final chocolate, it does play an essential role in the next step—fermentation.

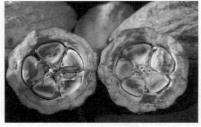

Step 3: Fermentation
The cacao beans, still covered with a sticky pulp, are covered with banana leaves and allowed to ferment. During the week or so that the cacao beans are allowed to ferment, the sugars in the pulp are converted to alcohol and organic acids and the beans develop the flavors and aromas characteristic of chocolate. The interior of the beans changes color during this time, turning a deep brown.

Step 4: Drying
The fully fermented beans must be dried or they will become moldy. During this phase, the cacao beans are reduced to about

half of their original weight. Typically, cacao beans are sun dried on bamboo mats. However, in rainy climates or during wet parts of the growing cycle, they may be taken indoors and dried using blowers that circulate warm air. But if the beans are dried too quickly, some of the fermentation processes are prematurely halted and the beans develop an acidic, bitter tang rather than a rich, desirable chocolate flavor.

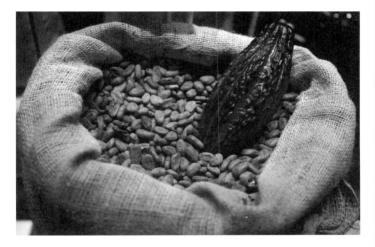

Step 5: Packing and shipping
The dried cacao beans are packaged in 200-pound sacks and then shipped, along with documentation of their varieties and origins, to central locations for inspection by cacao purchasers.

Step 6: Inspection and sales
Commercial lots of cacao beans are inspected by buyers, who are contracted to purchase the beans on behalf of chocolate producers around the world. Buyers randomly inspect the beans, cutting some of them open to assess their color and aroma and to ensure that proper fermentation has taken place. Buyers also verify that the beans are free of mold and other disease.

Step 7: Sorting and cleaning
During this first step of the manufacturing process, the bulk cacao beans are sorted and cleaned of any field-processing residue.

Step 8: Roasting
Cacao beans are roasted at temperatures of 250 degrees Fahrenheit or more. Like coffee beans, cacao beans only develop their rich flavors after a period of roasting. And like coffee, the flavor of chocolate is strongly influenced by how the beans are roasted. Intense roasting for as little as 30 minutes produces the strongest chocolate flavor, while slower roasting at lower temperatures produces more intricate flavors with complex floral notes. (Connoisseurs of fine chocolates, much like wine experts, can recognize and appreciate the subtle differences between chocolates derived from different varieties of cacao with different roasting times and temperatures.)

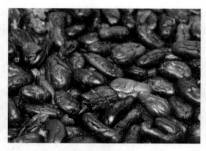

Step 9: Cracking and separating
When the roasted cacao beans have cooled, the outer shells are cracked open to expose the interior nutmeats (cacao nibs). Large fans blow away the shell fragments, after which the broken seed parts are winnowed through a series of graded sieves. At the end of this process, the cacao nibs contain a mixture of about 47 percent cocoa solids and 53 percent cocoa butter (vegetable fat). Until recently, cacao nibs were used only as an intermediate product in the chocolate-making process. However, some natural food purveyors now sell cacao nibs directly to consumers.

Step 10: Milling
The cacao nibs are passed through a series of grinders that mill the nibs into a liquefied paste called chocolate liquor (no relation to alcoholic liquor).

Step 11: Cocoa butter extraction
Some of the chocolate liquor is taken out of the production flow for the extraction of cocoa butter. Cocoa butter is extracted by subjecting the chocolate liquor to very high pressure; under intense pressure, the yellow liquid cocoa butter separates from the cocoa solids and oozes through screens into collection vessels. The extracted cocoa butter can then be added to other chocolate products or used in the preparation of various cosmetics and medicines. Cocoa butter is also used as the base for producing white chocolate (which contains no cocoa solids and is therefore, strictly speaking, not chocolate at all).

Step 12: Blending
The pure chocolate liquor, with its ratio of cocoa solids and cocoa butter intact, may now be blended with additional cocoa butter, milk, sweeteners and other flavors. (Additional cocoa butter is used to fine-tune the chocolate for optimal mouthfeel—the melt-in-your-mouth quality that makes chocolate so irresistible.) Once all the desired ingredients have been added, the mixture is churned into a coarse powder called crumb.

Step 13: Refining
The chocolate crumb is passed through a series of steel rollers to refine its texture. Longer refining times will yield a silkier texture, but overworking the chocolate can create an undesirable gummy texture.

Step 14: Conching
The refined chocolate crumb is massaged with special metal rollers shaped like conch shells. Conching, invented in 1879 by the Swiss chocolate maker Rudolphe Lindt, perfects the mixture of the elements in the crumb. It also aerates the mix, allowing residual moisture to escape into the air and producing a mellower, more refined chocolate flavor.

Step 15: Tempering
The chocolate is repeatedly warmed and cooled, ensuring that the

final chocolate product will have a glossy sheen and a consistent melting point. At a microscopic level, tempering creates a perfectly regular pattern of crystallization, enhancing the chocolate's mouthfeel. Expert chocolate chefs will sometimes temper chocolate by warming it and spreading it out over a cool slab of marble.

Step 16: Fabrication
At this stage, the tempered chocolate is ready to be made into its final form. Chocolate makers frequently use molds to give chocolate attractive shapes—from simple bars to beautiful forms like seashells and animals. Even seasonal favorites like chocolate Easter bunnies or Santa Claus figures can be molded in this way, as can hollow forms that are then filled with fruits, nuts, creams, jellies, ganache and other treats.

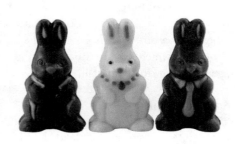

* * * *

As you can see, even the basic steps of chocolate making are quite complex. Of course, the possibilities do not end here. For example, the Dutch process, invented in the early nineteenth century by Dutch chemist Coenraad Johannes van Houten, yields a less bitter type of chocolate often used for baking and hot chocolate.

The Dutch process involves treating chocolate nibs with an alkalizing agent (usually potassium or sodium bicarbonate) before roasting. Dutched cocoa has a much darker color than unprocessed cocoa; however, if you're interested in the antioxidants and other potentially beneficial phytochemicals in chocolate, avoid Dutch-processed products—alkalization destroys these nutrients.

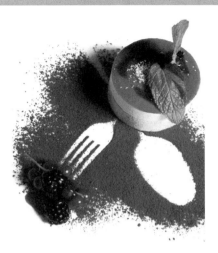

In recent years, some manufacturers have simplified the chocolate-making process and begun marketing raw chocolate products, which they claim have higher levels of beneficial antioxidants and other nutrients. These raw chocolate products are still quite rare and usually command extraordinary prices—as much as ten dollars for a 2-ounce bar! It seems a strange twist of economy, since raw chocolate requires so much less processing. Perhaps consumer demand will bring these astronomical prices down in the future. Until then, price-conscious consumers can enjoy the ever-increasing selection of chocolate as more and more artisanal varieties are introduced and the art of chocolate making, like the art of wine making, becomes more widely appreciated and enjoyed.

References

Biggs W. "Dark chocolate for your blood pressure?" *Journal Watch Women's Health.* 2007:1–1. Macht M, Dettmer D. "Everyday mood and emotions after eating a chocolate bar or an apple." *Appetite.* 2006; 46 (3): 332–6.

Macht M, Mueller J. "Immediate effects of chocolate on experimentally induced mood states." *Appetite.* 2007; May 23 (electronic publication ahead of print).

Mink PJ et al. "Flavonoid intake and cardiovascular disease mortality: a prospective study in postmenopausal women." *American Journal of Clinical Nutrition.* 2007; 85 (3): 895–909.

Mogelonsky M. "Premium chocolate confectionery—US—March 2007." *Mintel Market Research Reports.*

Morse G. "Decisions and desire." *Harvard Business Review.* 2006; 84 (1): 42, 44–51, 132.

Serafini, M et al. "Plasma antioxidants from chocolate." *Nature.* 2003; 424: 1013.

Smeets PA et al. "Effect of satiety on brain activation during chocolate tasting in men and women." *American Journal of Clinical Nutrition.* 2006; 83 (6): 1297–305.

Stat TY. "Hospital figures chocolate could be the best medicine." *Chicago Tribune.* July 29, 2007.

Stauth D. "Studies force new view on biology, nutritional action of flavonoids." *Medical News Today.* March 9, 2007. [Page number?]

Strecker M. "Chocolate toothpaste better than fluoride, researcher says." Tulane University, May 19, 2007. [Barbara: was this published in print format or did our did you access it online? If it was printed, we need publication name, date, issue, etc. If online, we need a URL.]

Taubert, D et al. "Chocolate and blood pressure in elderly individuals with isolated systolic hypertension." *Journal of the American Medical Association.* 2003; 290 (8): 1029–30.

Taubert D et al. "Effect of cocoa and tea intake on blood pressure: a meta-analysis [Review]." *Archives of Internal Medicine.* 2007; 167 (7): 626–634.

Taubert D et al. "Effects of low habitual intake on blood pressure and bioactive nitric oxide." *Journal of the American Medical Association.* 2007; 298: 49–60.

Vinson JA. "Chocolate is a powerful ex vivo and in vivo antioxidant, an antiatherosclerotic agent in an animal model, and a significant contributor to antioxidants in the European and American diets." *Journal of Agricultural and Food Chemistry.* 2006; 54 (21): 8071–6.